The Original Mediterranean Seafood Cookbook

An Entire Cookbook of Seafood Recipes

Joseph Bellisario

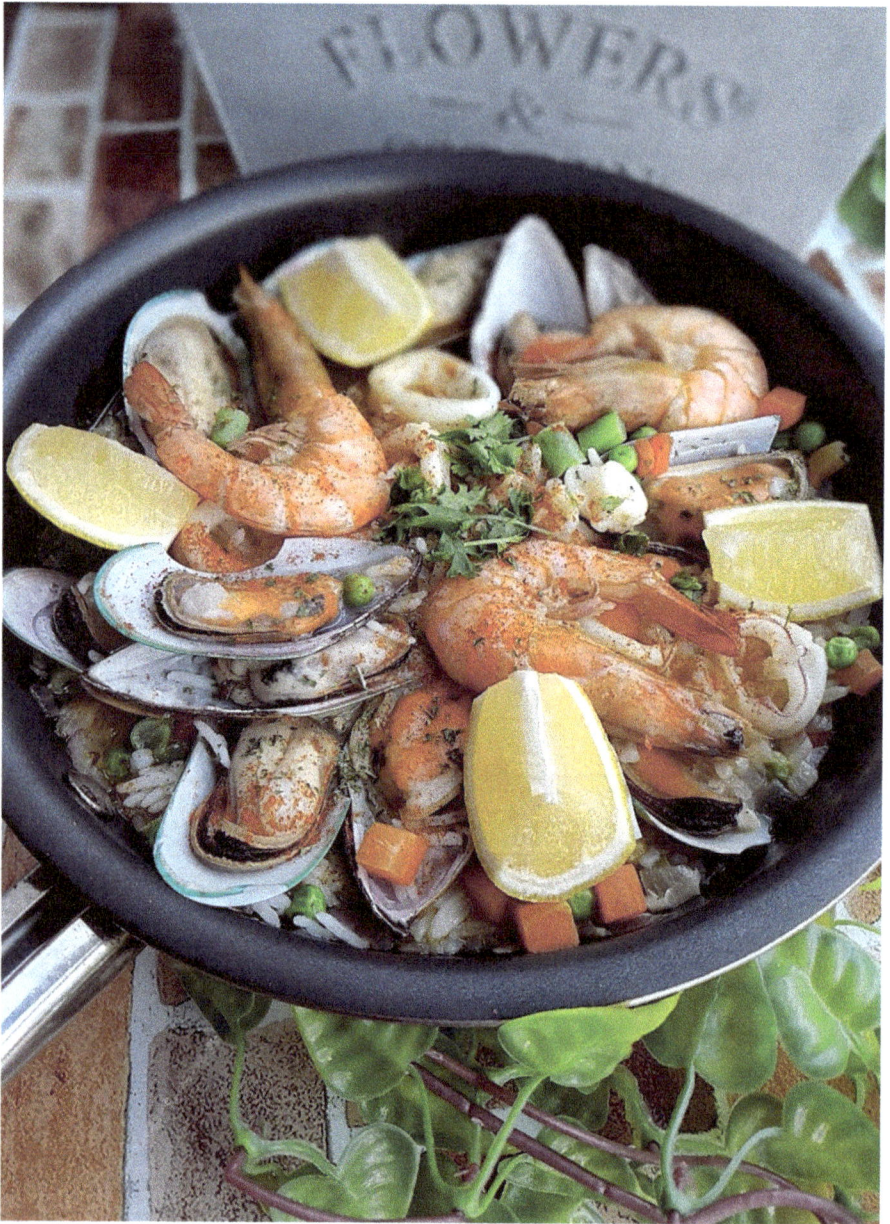

TABLE OF CONTENTS

4

Moroccan salmon

The Moroccan salmon derives its flavor and taste from variety of fruits and vegetables and herbs.

Mint and oranges are key healthy ingredients that elevate this Mediterranean Sea diet recipe.

Ingredients

- pinch of cayenne
- 2 salmon filets
- ½ teaspoon of cinnamon
- Orange zest
- ½ teaspoon of salt
- ¾ teaspoon of sugar
- 1 tablespoon of oil for searing
- ½ teaspoon of cumin

Directions

1. Preheat oven to 350°F.
2. In a small bowl, combine cinnamon together with the cumin, salt, sugar and cayenne .
3. Sprinkle over both sides of the salmon.

4. Heat oil in an oven proof skillet over medium temperature.
5. Sear salmon on both sides for 2 minutes each side.
6. Place in the warm oven to finish for 5 minutes.
7. Garnish with orange zest.
8. Serve and enjoy with Moroccan quinoa.

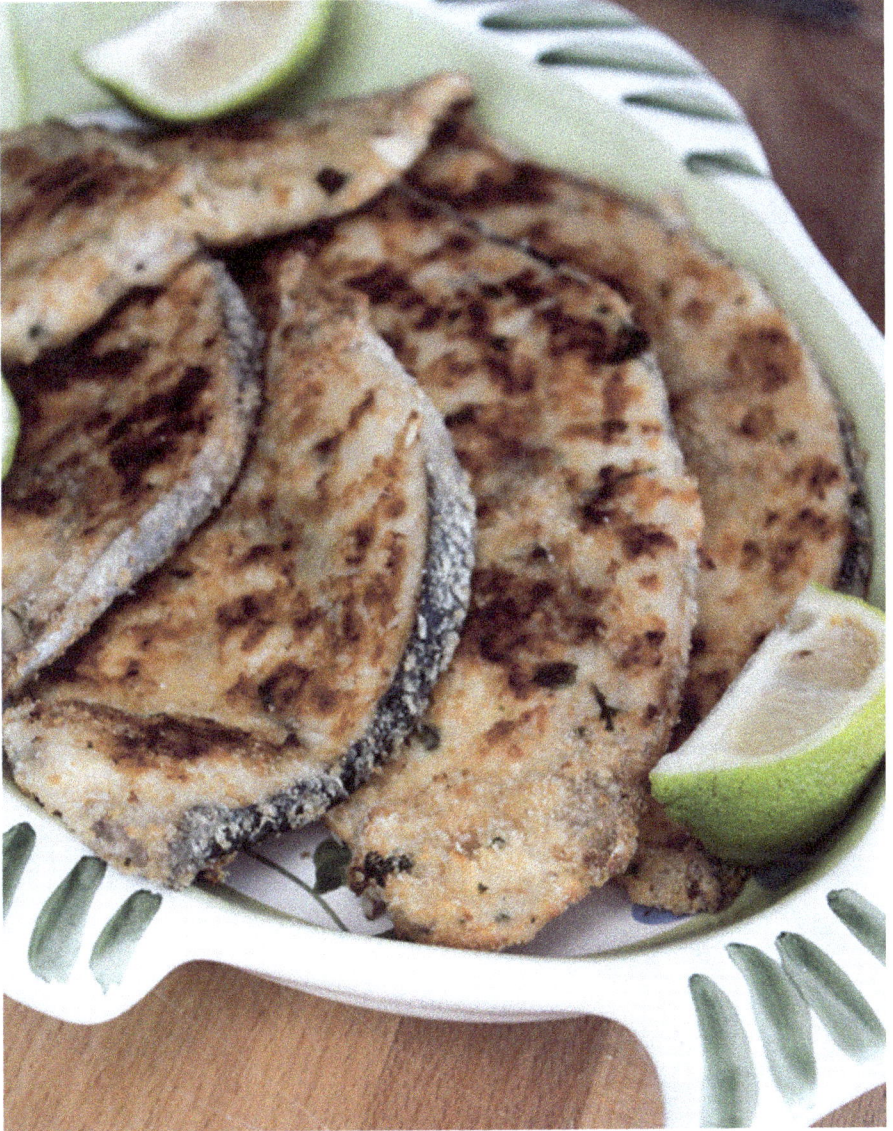

Pan seared salmon with chia seeds, fennel slaw and pickled onions

Ingredients

- ½ ounce of package dill
- ½ teaspoon of salt
- 3 tablespoon of lemon juice
- ¼ cup of thinly sliced sweet onion
- ½ teaspoon of dried mint, dill or tarragon
- ½ teaspoon of granulated garlic
- 1 Turkish cucumber
- 2 teaspoons of chia seeds
- Salt and pepper to taste
- 3 tablespoon of olive oil
- ½ lemon
- 2 6 ounces of wild Salmon
- 1 extra-large fennel bulb, thinly sliced

Directions

1. Place fennel bulb, cucumber, dill, olive oil, lemon juice, lemon juice, salt and pepper in a medium bowl, toss well. Set aside.

2. Brush the tops of salmon with olive oil .

3. Place   salt together with the pepper, dried herbs, granulated garlic, chia seeds in a small bowl, mix.

4. Coat the top of the fish liberally with the chia mixture, pressing it down with fingers.

5. Then, heat olive oil in a pan over medium heat.

6. Let the pan get hot enough, then add the fish with chia seed side down and pan sear for 4 minutes until golden.

7. Turnover, to keep crust intact and continue cooking until fish is cooked in 4 minutes.

8. Serve and enjoy with a squeeze of lemon juice on top.

Ceviche

Ceviche is quite a delicious fish recipe that features cucumber, tomatoes, chilies, cilantro, lime and even avocado.

As a result, the variety of vegetables makes this recipe a perfect Mediterranean Sea diet choice for any meal.

Ingredients

- 1 cup of diced cucumber
- ½ of a red onion, thinly sliced
- 1 pound of fresh fish- sea bass
- 1 fresh serrano chili pepper seeded
- 1 cup of grape
- 1 semi-firm avocado, diced
- 3 garlic cloves finely minced¼ teaspoon of black pepper
- ½ cup of fresh cilantro chopped
- 1 ½ teaspoon of kosher salt
- ¾ cup of fresh lime juice
- 1 tablespoon of olive oil

Directions

1. Place fish together with the onion, garlic, salt , fresh chilies, pepper, and lime juice in a shallow serving bowl , mix.
2. Transfer to a refrigerator to marinate for at 45 minutes.
3. Gently toss in the fresh cilantro with cucumber and tomato.
4. Drizzle with olive oil , mix.
5. Taste, and adjust accordingly.
6. Gently fold in the avocado at the end, after mixing everything.
7. Serve and enjoy.

Seared Hawaiian ono with honey soy glaze and pineapple salsa

Ingredients

- 1 teaspoon of finely minced or grated ginger root
- 1 mild red chili
- 2 lbs. of Fresh Ono cut into 6 pieces
- ⅓ cup of soy sauce
- ⅓ cup of honey
- 3 teaspoon of sliced ginger
- ⅛ teaspoon of kosher salt
- 2 garlic cloves
- ¼ cup of finely diced red onion
- 1 teaspoon of olive oil
- zest and juice of one small lime
- ½ cup of chopped cilantro
- Pineapple Ginger Salsa
- ½ pineapple, pealed cored, small diced
- 1 jalapeño- seeds removed, diced

Directions

1. Blend soy sauce together with the honey , garlic, sliced ginger, and olive oil in a blender until smooth.
2. Put the fish and marinade in a Ziploc bag for 20 minutes or longer.
3. Cut pineapple in half, saving top half for another use.
4. Slice and dice into ½ inch cubes, then place in a medium bowl.
5. Toss in the jalapeno, red chili, red onion, ginger root, cilantro, zest and juice and kosher salt.
6. Taste, and adjust accordingly.
7. Heat oil in a large heavy bottom skillet, over medium temperature.
8. When oil is hot enough, place in the fish, saving the marinade.
9. Sear the fish, on its sides, set aside.
10. Pour the remaining marinade into the skillet let boil briefly.
11. Strain and place in a small bowl.
12. Spoon over the fish, with a generous amount of pineapple salsa.
13. Serve and enjoy.

Sea base with cannellini bean stew

A combination of beans and fish is an incredible protein blast.

In 30 minutes, this Mediterranean Sea diet recipe will be just ready waiting for your bite.

Ingredients

- • ½ teaspoon of kosher salt
- 2 tablespoons of olive oil
- ¼ teaspoon of cracked pepper
- 1 medium onion, diced
- Oil, salt and pepper for fish
- 1 cup of peeled, diced carrot
- 4 cups of chicken stock
- 1 cup of diced celery
- Italian parsley for garnish
- 4 smashed and roughly chopped garlic cloves
- 2 cups of diced tomatoes
- 4 four-ounce of sea bass fillets
- 3 cups of cannellini beans
- 1 cup of water
- 2 tablespoons of fresh sage

Directions

1. In a medium heavy-bottomed pot, heat oil over medium heat.
2. Add onions, stir for 2 minutes.
3. Add carrots together with the celery and garlic, sauté over medium heat for 5 minutes, stirring occasionally.
4. Add canned beans with the 2 cups of stock, herbs, tomatoes, salt and pepper, let boil.
5. Lower the heat, cover, let simmer for 15 minutes.
6. Heat 2 tablespoons of olive oil in a skillet, over medium temperature.
7. Pat dry fish with paper towels.
8. Season generously with kosher salt and pepper.
9. Sear each side until a golden crust forms on the fish.
10. Lower the heat, let cook through.
11. Place the stew in a wide shallow dish topping with seared fish
12. Serve and enjoy garnished with fresh Italian parsley.

Authentic aguachile with shrimp

This Mediterranean Sea diet recipe is simple, yet flavorful and tasty appetizer similar to ceviche recipe.

Ingredients

- 1 serrano chili, sliced in half lengthwise
  - 1 teaspoon of kosher salt
- 2 large limes
- 1 cup of cilantro
- ½ cup of fresh lime juice
- Pinch of salt
- ¼ of a red onion, thinly sliced
- Splash of white vinegar
- 1 pound of raw shrimp
- Water
- 1 garlic clove
- 2 jalapeños, sliced in half lengthwise

Directions

1. Place the sliced shrimp in a shallow serving dish in one layer.
2. Squeeze lime to cover the shrimp, turning slightly pink.

3. Sprinkle with a little salt .
4. Cook the shrimp turning over as needed in the lime juice for 20 minutes.
5. Season the red onion with salt .
6. Pour just enough water to cover the onions, add a splash of white vinegar .
7. Combine lime juice, cilantro, jalapeno, chili, and kosher salt in a food processor, blend till smooth.
8. Pour the mixture over the shrimp and toss to coat.
9. Drain the onions and scatter them over, mixing slightly.
10. Refrigerate for 4 hours.
11. Taste, and adjust accordingly.
12. Serve and enjoy with tortilla chips.

Roasted mustard seed white fish with potato Brussel sprout hash

Ingredients

- 10 ounces of potatoes, thinly sliced
- 2 teaspoons of olive oil
- Salt and pepper to taste
- 1 large shallot, thinly sliced
- 1 tablespoon of olive oil
- 6 ounce filets of fish
- 4 teaspoons of whole grain mustard
- 8 ounces of Brussel Sprouts, thinly sliced
- Pinch of caraway seeds

Directions

1. Firstly, preheat your oven ready to 450°F.
2. Slice potatoes and shallots, toss with oil, salt and pepper in a mixing bowl.
3. Place on a parchment lined baking sheet in a single layer, let bake for 20 minutes.
4. Slice and place Brussel sprouts in the same oily bowl.
5. Toss, then, add a pinch of caraway seeds . Set aside.

6. Mix the whole grain mustard together with oil in a small bowl.

7. Season the fish with salt and pepper.

8. Divide the mustard mixture, then spoon over the fish.

9. When the potatoes have baked for 20 minutes, add the brussel sprouts, toss.

10. Make a spot for the fish, let bake for 12 minutes, until cooked through.

11. Divide the potato Brussel sprout hash among two bowls and top with the mustard glazed fish.

12. Serve and enjoy.

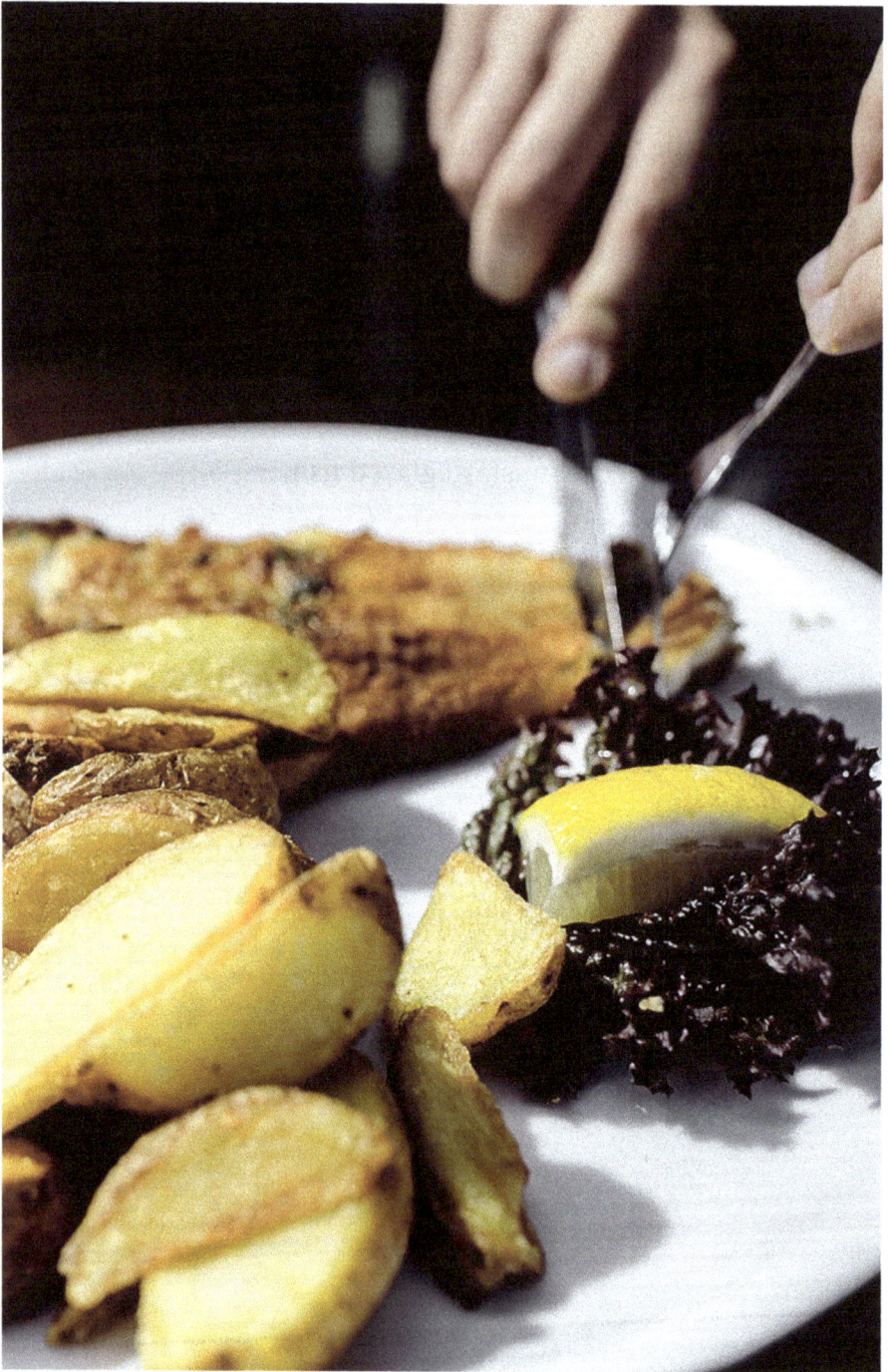

Pomegranate glazed mackerel with satsuma and fennel salad

Ingredients

- 4 mackerel fillets
- 40ml of runny honey
- 2 medium beetroots
- 1 tablespoon of pomegranate molasses
- 1 small red onion
- 1 teaspoon of runny honey
- 1 small fennel
- 40ml of pomegranate molasses
- 6 satsumas
- 1 bunch of fresh dill
- 4 tablespoons of extra virgin olive oil
- 1 lemon

Directions

1. Preheat the oven ready to 400°F.
2. Then, wrap each beetroot individually in foil, let roast for 45 minutes, let cool.
3. In a large bowl, combine the pomegranate molasses together with the honey and 40ml of satsuma, season.

4. Place the mackerel into the mixture, let marinate for 20 minutes.

5. Combine sliced satsuma with the red onion, fennel and beetroot. Set aside.

6. Also, combine the olive oil together with the lemon juice, molasses, and honey in a small bowl, whisk. Set aside for later.

7. Remove the mackerel fillets from the marinade and place on a baking tray lined with foil.

8. Transfer the marinade into a small saucepan, bring to the boil over a high heat for 5 minutes. Set aside for the glaze.

9. Preheat your grill to high, grill the fillets for 4 minutes.

10. Remove from the oven and brush with the glaze, then season.

11. Drizzle the vinaigrette over the salad and toss to combine.

12. Roughly chop and add the dill.

13. Serve and enjoy with the mackerel.

Coconut lemongrass scallops with lime

The coconut lemongrass scallop recipe is stuffed with herbs and lime zest for a healthy Mediterranean Sea diet.

Ingredients

- 4 tablespoons of white vinegar
- 1 can of coconut milk
- Kaffir lime leaves
- 1 stalk of fresh lemongrass, smashed
- 1 large lime zest and juice
- 1 ½ teaspoons of fish sauce
- Slices red chili
- 1 ¼ pound of large scallops
- 1 tablespoon coconut oil
- 1 shallot, diced
- Salt and pepper
- 8 leaves of fresh basil
- 2 thin slices ginger

Directions

1. Cook a small pot of rice on stove.
2. In a small saucepan, simmer, on low heat, shallot in vinegar, until vinegar reduces in 5 minutes.
3. Add coconut milk with smashed lemongrass, ½ of the lime zest, and ginger, let simmer on low heat for 5 minutes.
4. Stir in fish sauce and lime juice.
5. Taste, and adjust accordingly. Let rest and flavors infuse.
6. Rinse, pat dry scallops.
7. Then, season with salt and pepper.
8. In a skillet, heat coconut oil over medium heat.
9. When hot enough, add the scallops and sear each side for 3 minutes.
10. Divide rice between bowls, top with scallops, place flavorful lemongrass coconut sauce over the top.
11. Serve and enjoy.

Smoked salmon, avocado, and fennel salad

Ingredients

- 6 ounces of smoked salmon
- ⅓ cup of mayo
- 2 tablespoons capers
- 1/3 cup of sour cream
- 1 tablespoon of olive oil
- 1 avocado , sliced
- ¼ cup of thinly sliced red onion
- 2 tablespoons of lemon juice
- 2 garlic cloves-finely minced
- 1/3 cup of fresh dill, chopped
- Sunflower sprouts
- ¼ heaping teaspoon of salt
- ¼ teaspoon of fresh cracked pepper
- 1 head of butter lettuce
- 1 Turkish cucumber, sliced
- ½ a fennel bulb, thinly sliced

Directions

1. Combine mayo, sour cream, olive oil, lemon juice, garlic, salt and pepper in a bowl, whisk until smooth.
2. Add the dill, then mix. Set aside.
3. Place the lettuce together with the fennel bulb, smoked salmon, cucumber, red onion, and capers in a big bowl.
4. Toss, then add enough dressing to coat.
5. Divide the salad and garnish with avocado and sprinkle with salt and pepper.
6. Serve and enjoy.

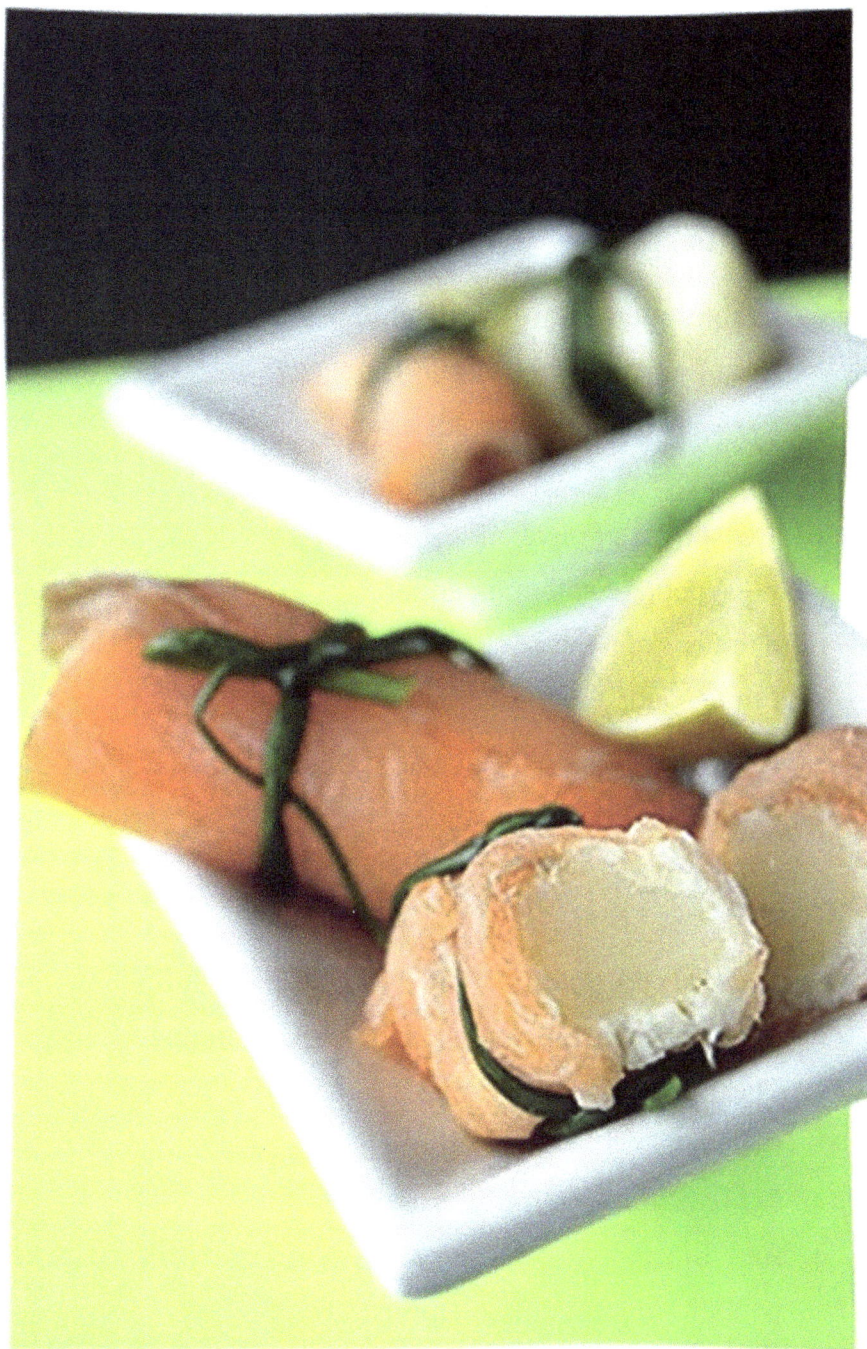

Dover sole with lemon, dill, and leeks

Ingredients

- 2 tablespoons of fresh dill, chopped
- 2 medium leeks, thinly sliced
- ⅛ teaspoon of kosher salt
- 10 ounces of dover sole
- 5teaspoons of olive oil
- 1 teaspoon of salt and pepper
- 8 ounces of baby potatoes
- 1 tablespoon of lemon juice
- Zest from ½ a lemon

Directions

1. Place sliced potatoes and leeks in a medium bowl and toss with olive oil, pepper, salt, and lemon zest.
2. Place on a parchment lined sheet-pan in a single layer in the oven.
3. Let bake for 20 minutes, tossing.
4. Add the fish to the same bowl, drizzle with oil, salt , pepper and remaining lemon zest.
5. Toss to coat all sides. Keep aside.

6. Combine dill, olive oil, lemon juice and kosher salt in a bowl.
7. Lay the fish over top of ready potatoes and return to the oven.
8. Let bake for 10 minutes.
9. Serve and enjoy.

Smoked salmon hand rolls with avocado

Ingredients

- 3 cups of calrose rice
- 2 cups of sprouts
- 2 packages nori sheets
- 2 tablespoons of seasoned rice wine vinegar
- Wasabi paste
- 2 teaspoon of toasted sesame seeds
- 16 ounces of smoked salmon
- 8 ounces of sliced mushrooms
- Soy sauce
- 1 tablespoon of oil
- 1 teaspoon of soy sauce
- 1 red bell pepper
- 1 cucumber, cut into strips
- 2 avocados , cut into strips

Directions

1. Bring rice to a boil, cover, and simmer on low for 20 minutes.

2. Place rice in a wood bowl , sprinkle with the seasoned rice vinegar .

3. Slice the rice and sprinkle with toasted sesame seeds and cover with a damp kitchen towel .

4. Sauté mushrooms in olive oil over medium heat.

5. Add sesame oil , cook for 2 more minutes.

6. Season with soy sauce .

7. Place bell pepper, cucumber and avocado in individual bowls.

8. Place the sprouts in a bowl and smoked salmon on a small platter

9. Place nori sheet horizontally.

10. Spread sushi rice on the left half of the sheet, align strips of veggies, diagonally. top with smoked salmon, mushrooms, and sprouts.

11. Serve and enjoy.

Baked cod recipe with garlic and lemon

Ingredients

- 3 tablespoon of olive oil
- 2 tablespoons of finely chopped preserved lemon
  - 1 teaspoon of kosher salt
- ½ cup of white wine
- ½ teaspoon of pepper
- 1 large bunch asparagus
- Zest from 1 lemon
- 1 large fennel bulb
- Cod
- Pinch salt and pepper
- ½ cup of chicken
- 1 large leek, white
- 4 cloves garlic, rough chopped
- 2 teaspoons of fresh thyme
- 1 tablespoons of fresh thyme

Directions

1. Preheat oven to 400°F.

2. Place cod in a bowl, drizzle with olive oil and sprinkle with salt and pepper, thyme, and zest.
3. Heat olive oil over medium heat.
4. Add fennel, sauté for 7 minutes, stir.
5. Add leeks and garlic, continue cooking, stirring.
6. Add preserved lemon with the fresh thyme, broth, and white wine.
7. Stir in salt and pepper and let simmer on low heat for 5 minutes.
8. Nestle in the fish in the pan, bake for 10 minutes.
9. Serve and enjoy.

White miso black cod

Ingredients

- 1/3 cup of sugar
- 3 tablespoons of sake
- 4 x 4 ounce pieces of Black Cod
- 1/3 cup of white miso paste
- 3 tablespoons of mirin

Directions

1. Bring the mirin and sake to a boil.
2. Whisk in the miso until dissolved.
3. • Add the sugar and cook over moderate heat, whisk.
4. Transfer the marinade to a large baking dish and let cool
5. Add the fish to the marinade and turn to coat.
6. Refrigerate overnight.
7. Preheat your oven ready to 400°F.
8. Heat a small oil, the wipe the marinade off the fish.
9. Place the fish, skin side up, in the skillet, sear until golden.
10. Turnover, crisp up the skin for 3 minutes.
11. Roast for 10 more minutes.
12. Serve and enjoy.

Baked salmon recipe with asparagus and yogurt dill sauce

Ingredients

- 1 large bunch asparagus
- 1 ¼ lb. of wild king salmon filet
- 2 tablespoons olive oil
- Squeeze of lemon to taste
- Salt and pepper to taste
- Lemon zest from one lemon
- ½ cup of plain whole fat yogurt
- ¼ cup of chopped parsley
- 1 tablespoon olive oil
- 1 garlic clove, finely minced
- Lemon zest
- Cracked pepper to taste
- ¼ teaspoon salt
- ¼ cup of chopped dill

Directions

1. Preheat your oven ready to 375°F.
2. Toss asparagus with a drizzle of olive oil .
3. Season and place on a parchment -lined sheet pan .

4. Place the salmon in the middle of the asparagus and drizzle with olive oil

5. Season with salt and pepper, lemon zest.

6. Bake in the oven for 20 minutes or more.

7. Combine yogurt, olive oil, garlic, lemon zest, salt, dill, and pepper in a small bowl, whisk.

8. Serve and enjoy.

Smoked mackerel pate with griddled toast and cress salad

Ingredients

- Extra virgin olive oil
- 400g of smoked mackerel
- 2 sticks of celery
- 200g of light cream cheese
- 6 slices of good bread
- 3 lemons
- 1 small bunch of fresh flat-leaf parsley
- 2 small punnets of cress

Directions

1. Break up the mackerel is a blender or food processor slightly.
2. Add the cream cheese with bit of parsley leaves, zest and most of the juice of 1 lemon and a few leaves of parsley. Blend until creamy pate. Season.
3. Toss the snipped cress, celery leaves, celery sticks, and the remaining parsley leaves.
4. Dress with a good squeeze of lemon juice, a splash of extra virgin olive oil, and some salt and pepper.

5. Heat a griddle pan till hot.
6. Add the bread, in batches, press down with a frying pan to squash against the griddle ridges.
7. Toast for 1 minute, turning halfway.
8. Serve and enjoy with lemon wedges and herb salad.

Lemony prawn courgette

Ingredients

- 20g of pine nuts
- ½ a fresh red chili
- 1 lemon
- 120 g ripe cherry tomatoes
- 140g of large raw peeled prawns
- Extra virgin olive oil
- 3 medium courgettes
- 1 clove of garlic

Directions

1. Preheat the oven to 400°F.
2. Place the prawns in a mixing bowl.
3. Squeeze in half the juice of lemon.
4. Season with sea salt and black pepper.
5. Stir well, then leave to one side to mingle flavors.
6. Put the cherry tomatoes on a small baking tray, let roast in the hot oven for 7 minutes.
7. Place a frying pan over a medium-high heat.
8. Add a drizzle of olive oil, then place in the sliced garlic with chili and fry, once golden, add the prawns, let cook for more 3 minutes, turning regularly.

9. Place the courgette, cherry tomatoes, and lemon juice in the pan, let cook for 1 minute, tossing often.
10. Toast the pine nuts in a dry pan until golden, then lightly crush.
11. Divide among plates, scatter over the crushed pine nuts, then drizzle over a little olive oil.
12. Serve and enjoy.

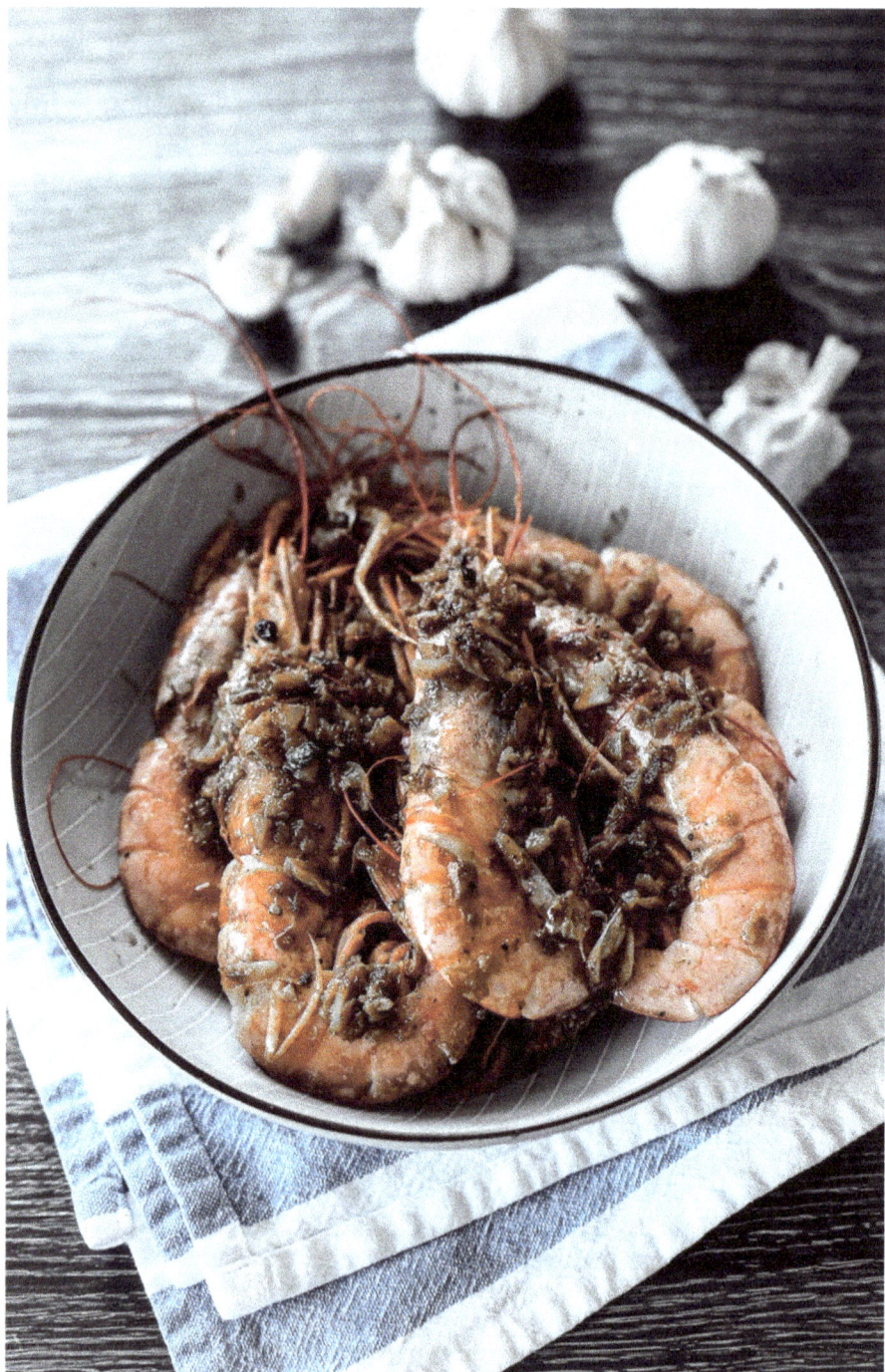

Grilled salmon with herby quinoa

Ingredients

- 4 salmon fillets, skin on
- 160g of ready to eat quinoa
- Extra virgin olive oil
- 2 lemons
- 4 tablespoons of natural yoghurt
- 2 courgettes
- 1 bulb of fennel
- 1 bunch of mixed fresh soft herbs

Directions

1. Begin by cooking the quinoa according to the packet Directions.
2. Squeeze over the juice of half a lemon.
3. Season with a pinch of sea salt and black pepper, set aside.
4. Preheat a griddle pan to high.
5. Griddle the courgette strips for 2 minutes on each side.
6. Place sliced fennel, herb leaves, lemon juice a bowl, stir through the quinoa, season.

7. Squeeze the remaining lemon juice into a small bowl, then add the yoghurt with olive oil, stir to combine.
8. Season with salt and pepper to taste.
9. Season and rub a little olive oil all over the salmon fillets, let cook on the hot griddle for 4 minutes each side.
10. Pile the quinoa on a plate and arrange the griddled courgette, lemony fennel on top, with flakes of salmon.
11. Serve and enjoy.

Keralan fish curry

Ingredients

- 1 teaspoon of turmeric
- 6 shallots
- 1 x 400g tin of light coconut milk
- 4 cloves of garlic
- 2.5cm piece of ginger
- 1 tablespoon of chili powder
- 1 x 400g tin of chopped tomatoes
- 1 fresh green chili
- 750g of firm white fish
- A few sprigs of fresh coriander
- Groundnut oil
- 1 teaspoon of mustard seeds
- 20 curry leaves

Directions

1. Heat groundnut oil, then add the mustard seeds together with the curry leaves, cook until the seeds begin to pop.
2. Add the shallot together with the garlic, ginger, and chili, cook on a medium heat for 5 minutes.
3. Mix the chili powder and turmeric with a splash of water, stir into the pan.

4. Fry for 1 minute, add the fish together with the coconut milk and tomatoes.
5. Season, bring to the boil, let simmer for 20 minutes.
6. Scatter the coriander leaves over the dish.
7. Serve and enjoy with basmati rice.

Baked sole goujons

Ingredients

- 2 large handfuls of breadcrumbs
- 2 large free-range eggs
- Olive oil
- 50g of plain flour
- 1 tablespoon of sweet smoked paprika
- 450 g lemon sole fillets

Directions

1. Preheat the oven to 410°F.
2. Cut the fish into finger-width strips.
3. Season the flour and place on a plate.
4. Crack the eggs into a shallow bowl, lightly beat.
5. Mix the paprika with the breadcrumbs on a separate plate.
6. Coat the fish goujons with the seasoned flour, dipping them in the eggs, then coating with the breadcrumbs.
7. Place them on the oiled tray, let bake until golden.
8. Serve and enjoy best with tartare sauce.

Prawn and courgette spaghetti

Ingredients

- 600g of raw peeled prawns
- 2 cloves of garlic
- 3 green courgettes
- 2 fresh red chilies
- ½ lemon
- Parmesan cheese
- 1 bunch of fresh dill
- 2 yellow courgettes
- 500g of dried spaghetti
- 1 large knob of unsalted butter
- Extra virgin olive oil

Directions

1. Cook the pasta according to the packet Directions.
2. Melt the butter with a splash of oil in a large frying pan on a medium heat.
3. Add the courgettes, let cook until slightly browned.
4. Add the garlic, chili, and prawns, cook until the prawns are cooked through.
5. Remove, squeeze over the lemon juice.
6. Drain the pasta, reserving a little cooking water.

7. Add the pasta to the frying pan and tossing with the courgettes and prawns.
8. Stir in the dill.
9. Season, and adjust accordingly.
10. Serve and enjoy with a grating of Parmesan.

Green tea roasted salmon

Ingredients

- 1 fresh red chili
- 150g of brown rice
- 1 x 3cm piece of ginger
- 1 x 500g of salmon tail, skin on, scaled, bone in
- Low-salt soy sauce
- ½ a punnet of cress
- 1 green tea bag
- 1 teaspoon of sesame seeds
- Sesame oil
- 1 clove of garlic
- 320g of mixed salad vegetables
- 1 small ripe mango
- 1 lime

Directions

1. Preheat your oven to 350°F.
2. Then, cook the rice according to package Directions, drain.
3. Score the salmon skin at 2cm intervals.
4. Season with sea salt and black pepper and the green teabag contents.

5. Rub all over with 1 teaspoon of sesame oil, getting well into the cuts.

6. Poke a slice of garlic into each cut.

7. Let bake for 25 minutes.

8. Slice mango flesh into bowl squeezing all the juice, and lime juice with all the vegetables.

9. Season with soy sauce.

10. Add the chili, then toss with the vegetables and mango.

11. Place matchstick ginger, put into a frying pan on a medium heat with 1 teaspoon of sesame oil and seeds.

12. Fry until starting to crisp up, tossing regularly.

13. Stir in the rice.

14. Serve and enjoy with the salmon and rice.

Prawn and papaya salad

Ingredients

- ½ a bunch of fresh basil
- 4 spring onions
- 50g of unsalted peanuts
- Runny honey
- 3 cloves of garlic
- ½ a bunch of fresh coriander
- 400g of peeled prawns
- 1 cucumber
- 4 ripe tomatoes
- 650g of green papaya
- Groundnut oil
- 2 fresh red chilies
- 3 limes
- 3 tablespoons of fish sauce

Directions

1. Firstly, toast the peanuts in a large dry frying pan over a medium-high heat
2. Transfer to a bowl and set aside.
3. Return the frying pan to a medium-high heat with 1 tablespoon of oil and the garlic.

4. Fry briefly, then stir in the whole prawns, let fry until turning pink, place in then chopped prawns.

5. Cook for 1 minute, stir in the tomatoes, continue to cook for 3 minutes.

6. Remove, let cool.

7. Add garlic with toasted peanuts into a pestle and mortar, pound to a rough paste.

8. Add in lime juice, fish sauce, honey, then mix well.

9. Add halved cucumber, shredded green papaya to the dressing.

10. Add spring onions, chopped basil leaves, and coriander leaves to the bowl.

11. Add the cooled prawn mixture and toss well.

12. Roughly chop and scatter over the remaining peanuts.

13. Serve and enjoy with lime wedges.

Prawn salad with chili and white cabbage

Ingredients

- Fresh chervil
- Extra virgin olive oil
- 3 handfuls of fresh, raw, small shelled prawns
- 3 lemons, juice of plus the finely grated zest of ½ a lemon
- 1 red chili, seeded and finely sliced
- ½ white cabbage, finely shredded

Directions

1. Put the prawns into a shallow dish.
2. Squeeze over the juice of 2 lemons, toss slightly to coat, let marinate for 20 minutes. Drain any excess juice.
3. Mix the chili with the cabbage.
4. Add grated lemon zest with the marinated prawns, a splash of olive oil, and the juice of remaining lemon.
5. Toss gently together with the chervil.
6. Season with salt and freshly ground black pepper.
7. Serve and enjoy.

Roasted cod with pancetta and pea mash

Ingredients

- Extra virgin olive oil
- 4 thick pieces of cod fillet
- ½ a bunch of fresh mint
- 1 small knob of butter
- 8 thin slices of pancetta
- 60g of rocket
- 2 lemons
- 1 splash of milk
- 500g of potatoes
- 300g of frozen garden peas
- ½ a fresh red chili

Directions

1. Preheat your oven to 400°F.
2. Season the cod with sea salt and black pepper.
3. Then, place on an oiled baking tray, lay 2 slices of pancetta over the top of each fillet.
4. Place 4 halved lemons on the tray next to the fish.
5. Let roast in the preheated oven for 15 minutes.

6. Cook the quartered potatoes until soft in boiling salted water.

7. Cook the peas according to packet Directions, drain.

8. Blend the peas in a food processor.

9. Drain the potatoes and mash with butter, hot milk, salt and pepper, whisk the peas and the red chili.

10. Put the rocket in a mixing bowl, with the mint leaves, toss together.

11. Serve each piece of cod on a dollop of pea and potato mash.

12. Enjoy.

Fish in crazy water

Ingredients

- 150g of white wine
- 2 spring onions
- 2 x 350g of whole round fish
- 1 lemon
- ½ a bulb of fennel
- 1 carrot
- 200g of ripe mixed-color cherry tomatoes
- Extra virgin olive oil
- 3 cloves of garlic
- 1 bunch of mixed fresh soft herbs
- ½ of a fresh red chili
- 10 mixed olives
- Olive oil

Directions

1. Put a large frying pan on a high heat with 1 tablespoon of olive oil.
2. Stir in the onions together with the fennel and carrot.
3. After a short while, add the tomatoes, with the garlic, chili, and olives. Toss regularly for 2 minutes.

4. Lay the fish on top of the vegetables, then the herbs into the cavities, then pour over the wine.
5. Add about 300ml of water, cover, let boil on a high heat for 8 minutes
6. Pick the remaining herb leaves, finely grate the lemon zest over them, mix together.
7. Uncover the fish, let baste with its juices for 1 minute.
8. Remove to a plate, spoon over the vegetables, and juices, drizzle with extra virgin olive oil.
9. Scatter over the lemony herbs.
10. Serve and enjoy.

Baked tiella rice

Ingredients

- 500g of long-grain rice
- 300g of potatoes
- 750g of mussels
- 400ml of Prosecco
- 1 onion
- 1 clove of garlic
- 1 bunch of fresh flat-leaf parsley
- 2 sticks of celery
- 400g of ripe cherry tomatoes
- 1 courgette
- 60g of Parmesan cheese
- Extra virgin olive oil

Directions

1. Preheat the oven to 400°F.
2. Place quartered potatoes in an ovenproof earthenware pot.
3. Add onion, garlic, tomatoes, parsley, and celery to the pot.
4. Place in the Parmesan, and pour in the Prosecco and 8 tablespoons of olive oil.

5. Add the rice, season with sea salt and black pepper, then mix.
6. Place the mussels into a really hot pan, cover, and steam for 4 minutes until they open.
7. Remove the mussel shells.
8. Stir the mussels and any juices into the pot, then layer the courgette on top like a lid, grate over the remaining Parmesan.
9. Place on a high heat, and as soon as it starts to bubble, transfer to the oven for 45 minutes.
10. Let rest, serve and enjoy.

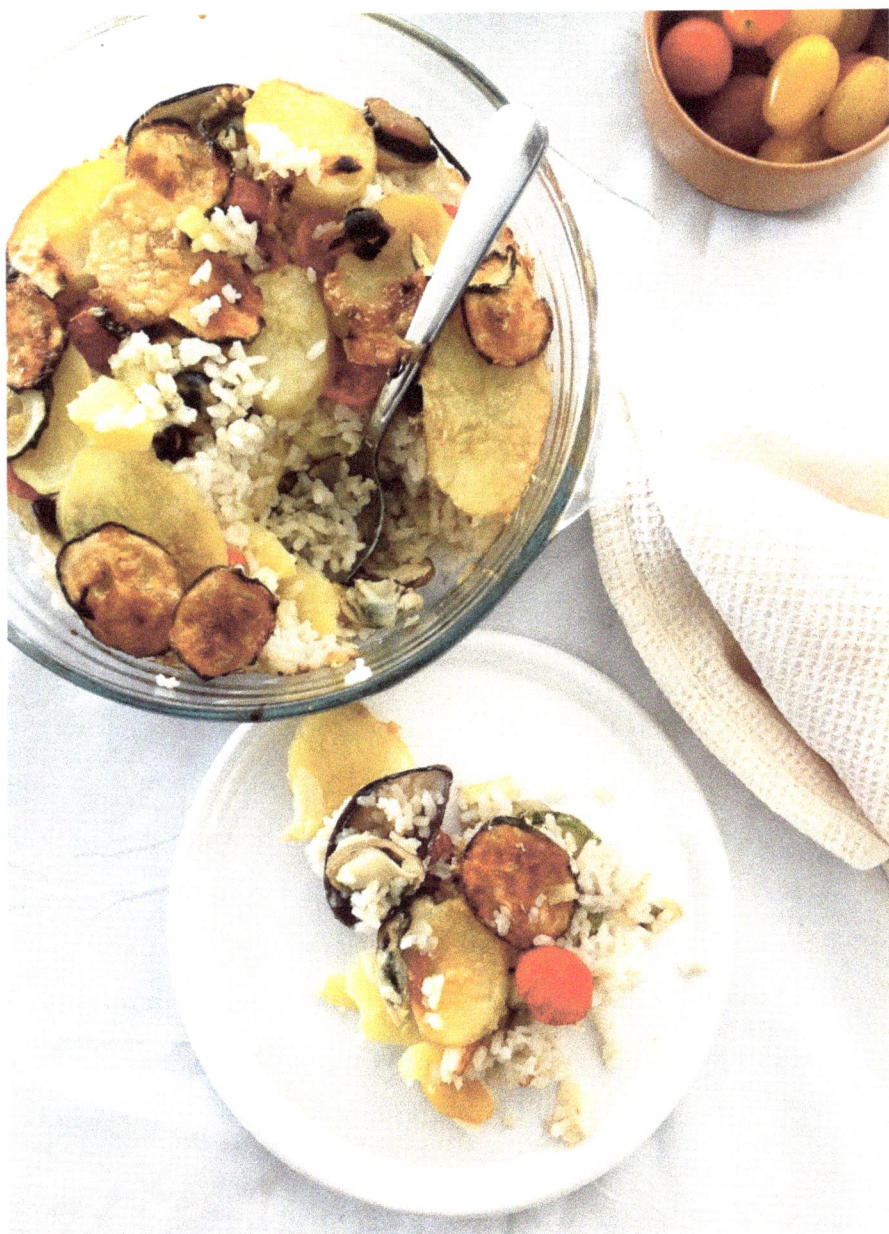

Smoked salmon blinis

Ingredients

- 1 cup of semi-skimmed milk
- 1 cup of self-rising flour
- Unsalted butter
- 1 large egg
- Olive oil

Directions

1. Place the flour with a pinch of sea salt in a large mixing bowl.
2. Make a well in the center, then, crack in the egg with 1 tablespoon of olive oil, beat into the flour.
3. Gently whisk in the milk until smooth batter forms.
4. Put a large non-stick frying pan on a medium heat.
5. Add 1 small knob of butter to melt.
6. Once melted, add tablespoons of batter to the pan.
7. Let, cook for 1 minute on each side, flipping over when they turn golden on the bottom.
8. Transfer the cooked blinis to a plate.
9. Then, continue with the remaining batter until it is all used up.
10. Serve and enjoy with combos.

Potted shrimp and crab

Ingredients

- 170g of white crabmeat
- 1 lemon
- 250g of unsalted butter
- ½ a bunch of fresh dill
- 1 whole nutmeg
- 180g of brown shrimp

Directions

1. Start by placing 100g of the butter into a pan over a medium heat for 10 minutes.
2. Strain the liquid into a separate bowl, let cool, and discard the leftover milky liquid.
3. Melt the remaining butter in a pan over a low heat, let cool briefly.
4. Chop and add stalks of dill with shrimp and crab into a bowl.
5. Grate half the lemon zest into the bowl, then squeeze in half the juice.
6. Grate in a little nutmeg, pour in the melted butter.
7. Then, season with sea salt and white pepper.

8. Spoon into a serving bowl, topping with the clarified butter, and scattered with the rest of the dill.
9. Refrigerate for 2 hours.
10. Serve and enjoy with crunchy radishes.

Prawn cocktail

Ingredients

- 1 swig of brandy
- 100g of mixed white and brown crabmeat
- Olive oil
- ½ a clove of garlic
- Cayenne pepper
- 1 small punnet of salad cress
- 1 heaped teaspoon of ketchup
- 8 unpeeled, large, raw tiger prawns
- ¼ of an iceberg lettuce
- 4 tablespoons of mayonnaise
- 50g of brown shrimps
- ¼ of a cucumber
- 2 ripe tomatoes
- 1 sprig of fresh mint
- 50g of peeled little prawns
- Lemon

Directions

1. Heat olive oil in a pan over a high heat.
2. Add crushed garlic, 1 pinch of cayenne pepper, and the tiger prawns.

3. Toss 4 minutes, or till cooked through.

4. Remove, and set aside.

5. Then, combine the lemon juice together with the remaining ingredients in a bowl, keep aside.

6. Layer sliced cucumber, shredded lettuce, mint leaves, and diced tomatoes in the bowl with most of the cress.

7. Add the peeled prawns, then, dollop with Marie rose sauce, finish with crabmeat, shrimps.

8. Add a pinch of cayenne pepper and hang a hot prawn on the side of the bowl.

9. Serve and enjoy with lemon wedges squeezed over.

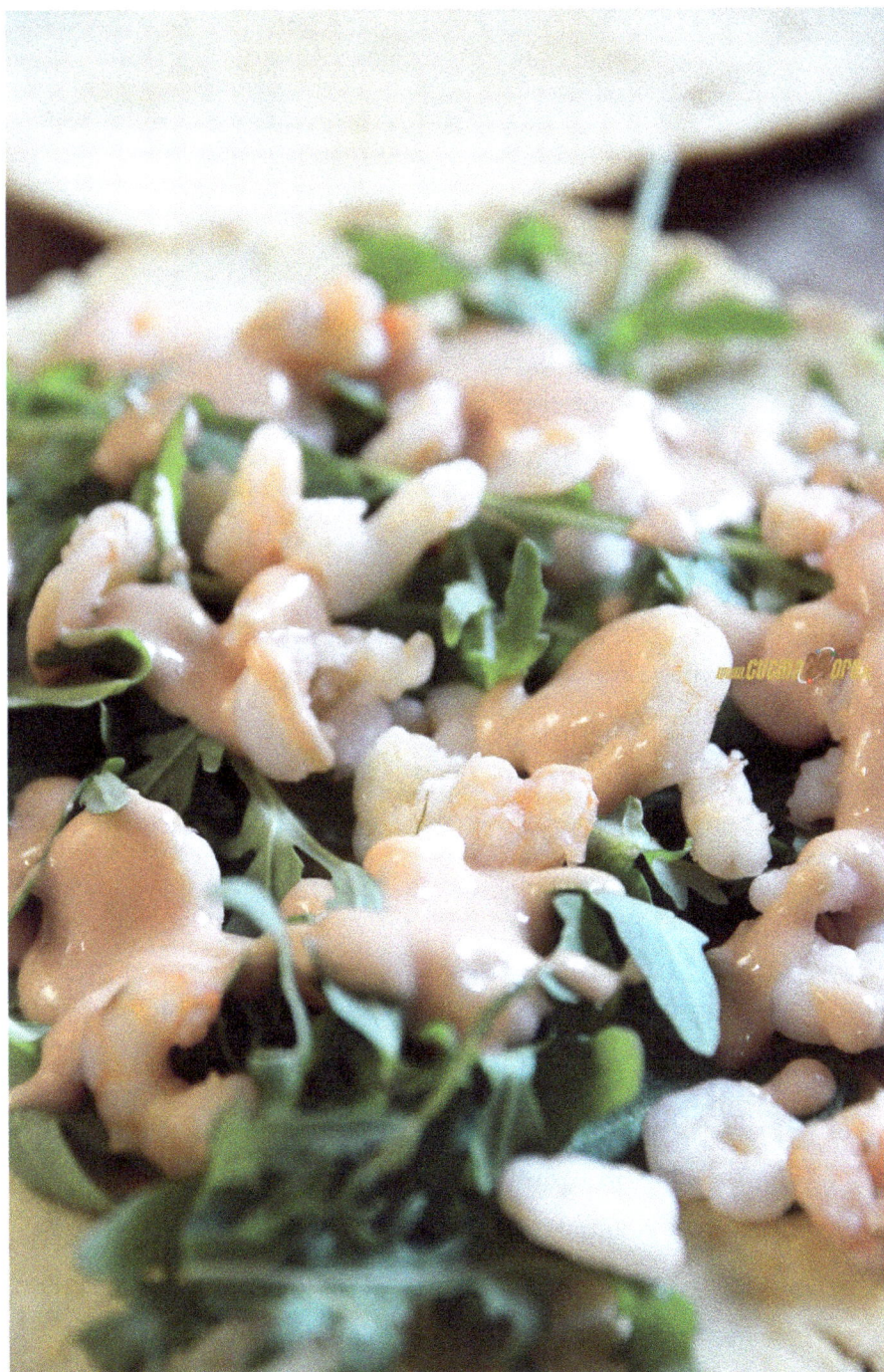

Cantonese-style steamed oyster

Ingredients

- 1 tablespoon of light soy sauce
- 16 large oysters, shells intact
- 2 fresh red chilies
- 1 teaspoon of chili bean sauce
- A few sprigs of fresh coriander
- 3 spring onions
- 3 tablespoons of groundnut oil
- 5cm piece of ginger
- 2 tablespoons of dark soy sauce
- 2 cloves of garlic
- 1 tablespoon of Shaoxing rice wine

Directions

1. Clean and divide the oyster between 2 heatproof plates.
2. Then, set up a steamer, fill with 5cm water.
3. Bring to the boil over a high heat.
4. Place 1 plate of oysters in the steamer covered.
5. Lower the heat, steam the oysters gently for 5 minutes.
6. Combine spring onions (shredded), chopped ginger, garlic, and chili with all the other ingredients apart from oil and coriander, add in a heatproof bowl.

7. Heat a large frying pan over a high heat until hot.
8. Add the olive oil until slightly smoking, then pour it over the sauce.
9. Remove the first batch of oysters from the steamer. stirs.
10. Remove the top shells of the oysters and drizzle a bit of sauce over each one.
11. Serve and enjoy with coriander leaves.

Brown shrimp on the toast

Ingredients

- 100ml of cider
- 1 knob of unsalted butter
- 4 slices of bread
- 200g of brown shrimps

Directions

1. Firstly, melt the butter in a pan over medium heat.
2. Then, add the shrimps.
3. Pour in the cider and bring to the boil.
4. Then, lower the heat, let simmer for 3 minutes, or until the cider has reduced.
5. Season with pepper.
6. Toast your bread, then top with the shrimps.
7. Serve and enjoy.

Lobster burger

Ingredients

- 2 ripe tomatoes
- 800g of cooked lobsters
- Olive oil
- 1 heaped teaspoon of Dijon mustard
- ½ a fresh red chili
- 4 thin rashers of smoked streaky bacon
- Red wine vinegar
- 4 burger buns
- 1 clove of garlic
- 1 red onion
- Tomato ketchup
- Mayonnaise
- Extra virgin olive oil
- 1 lemon
- 1 handful of watercress
- 1 soft round lettuce

Directions

1. Grate the tomatoes to a slurry on both sides, discarding the seeds and skin.
2. Grate in the chili, season well.

3. Then, add olive oil, a swig of vinegar, and stir in bit of fresh herbs.
4. Slice the lobster after twisting off the tails.
5. Leave the shell on.
6. Toss the chunks in olive oil, sea salt, black pepper, and mustard.
7. Let barbecue for 3 minutes on each side until cooked. Peel.
8. Also, barbecue the bacon, turning frequently till golden and crispy.
9. Toast the buns at the same time, then lay the bottom halves on a nice board.
10. Rub garlic over each side of halved buns.
11. Drizzle with oil, then add a tiny blob of ketchup, with bit of mayo and a squeeze of lemon juice.
12. Place the lettuce leaves, one onto each bun with a wodge of watercress.
13. Top with the lobster and salsa, then, crumble over the bacon.
14. Scatter over some sliced red onion, topping with the bun lid.
15. Secure the burgers with skewers.
16. Serve and enjoy.

Grilled lobster rolls

Ingredients

- 2 tablespoons of mayonnaise
- 85g of butter
- 6 submarine rolls
- 1 stick of celery
- ½ of an iceberg lettuce
- 500g of cooked lobster meat

Directions

1. Preheat a griddle pan until really hot.
2. Butter the rolls on both sides and grill until toasted on both sides and lightly charred.
3. Combine the celery, chopped lobster meat with the mayonnaise.
4. Season with sea salt and black pepper to taste.
5. Open warm grilled buns, shred and pile the lettuce inside each one.
6. Then, top with the lobster mixture.
7. Serve and enjoy right away.

Charred prawns in sweet aubergine sauce

Ingredients

- 2 aubergines
- 4 cloves of garlic
- Olive oil
- 2 large bunches of fresh basil
- 1kg of ripe tomatoes
- 1 teaspoon of dried oregano
- 2 fresh red chilies
- 3 tablespoons of red wine vinegar
- 16 king prawns

Directions

1. Combine garlic, basil leaves, chilies, red wine vinegar, olive oil, and seasoning in a blender, process to a paste.
2. Remove the prawn shells, then, cut along the back of each, and open up like a book.
3. Place into a bowl with basil paste, mix to coat.
4. Cover the bowl with Clingfilm, let marinate in the fridge for overnight.

5. Score a cross in the top of each tomato, place in a large bowl and cover with boiling water.
6. Drain the tomatoes, peel the skins, chop the flesh. Set aside.
7. Place a saucepan over a medium heat, add olive oil.
8. Add aubergines and fry for 10 minutes, stirring frequently.
9. Add the remaining chili, garlic, oregano, and basil stalk into the pan, fry briefly, stir in the tomatoes.
10. Add a few splashes of water, let simmer over low heat for about 30 minutes.
11. Place a griddle pan over a high heat.
12. Once hot enough, cook the prawns for 2 minutes on each side.
13. Drop the prawns into the sauce.
14. Stir the remaining basil leaves into the sauce.
15. Serve and enjoy.

Spicy prawn curry with quick Pilau rice

Ingredients

- 1 teaspoon of cumin seeds
- 1 small red onion
- 1 teaspoon of unsalted butter
- ½ a bunch of fresh coriander
- 5cm piece of ginger
- 1 onion
- 1 fresh green chili
- ½ mug of basmati rice
- olive oil
- 1 teaspoon of mustard seeds
- vegetable oil
- Turmeric
- 2 ripe tomatoes
- 200g of raw king prawns, shells on
- 1 fresh bay leaf
- 100ml of light coconut milk
- 3 cardamom pods
- 4 cloves

Directions

1. Heat 1 tablespoon of olive oil over a medium heat.
2. Add the red onion together with the coriander stalks, and dried spices, then fry for 1 minute.
3. Add the chopped ginger with the green chili, then cook for a further 5 minutes, stirring occasionally.
4. Add onion with vegetable oil and butter to a pan over a medium heat.
5. Let cook for 5 minutes, then, place a kettle of water on to boil.
6. Sprinkle in the spices, let cook for 1 minute.
7. Raise the heat, then, add the rice, stir well, add water twice the size of the rice mug, cook over reduced heat with a pinch of salt.
8. Simmer for 15 minutes over a low heat, or until the water has been absorbed.
9. Add the fresh tomatoes to the spiced onions with a splash of boiling water.
10. Bring to the boil, season, then simmer for 5 minutes.
11. Stir in the prawns together with the coconut milk, let cook for 5 minutes.
12. Fluff, serve and enjoy with the curry and scattering the coriander leaves on top.

Clams casino

Ingredients

- 1 knob of unsalted butter
- 10 large cherrystone clams
- 1 lemon
- 4 large cloves of garlic
- 200g of fresh white breadcrumbs
- ½ a bunch of fresh thyme
- Extra virgin olive oil
- 4 jarred red peppers
- 8 rashers of smoked streaky bacon

Directions

1. Preheat the grill to high.
2. Place a deep pan over a high heat.
3. Add the clams with a splash of water, cover.
4. Let cook over a high heat, shaking now and then, until all the clams have opened, let cool on a tray.
5. Snip each bacon rasher into 3, place the pieces in a non-stick frying pan.
6. Cook over a medium heat until the bacon is just starting to crisp.

7. Lift the pieces of bacon out of the pan onto a plate, return the pan to the heat.

8. Add the butter together with the garlic and thyme, then add the breadcrumbs when sizzling.

9. Let fry for 3 minutes, stirring.

10. Season with sea salt and black pepper. Remove, let cool.

11. Remove the clams from the shells, chop into quarters.

12. Place into a bowl, then add a squeeze of lemon juice, a drizzle of extra virgin olive oil, and a pinch of seasoning.

13. Rinse the shells, spread out on a large roasting tray.

14. Place a few pepper strips into each shell, then, bit of breadcrumbs.

15. Nestle a couple of clam quarters in each one and cover with more crumbs.

16. Top with a piece of bacon and drizzle extra virgin olive oil.

17. Place the tray on a low shelf under the hot grill for 5 minutes.

18. Serve and enjoy with the remaining lemon wedges squeezed over.

Boiled prawn wontons with chili dressing

Ingredients

- 20ml of light soy sauce
- 225g of raw prawns
- 1 teaspoon of dried chili flakes
- 1 spring onion
- 40ml of vegetable oil
- 1cm piece of ginger
- 20ml of rice wine vinegar
- 1 tablespoon of Sichuan pepper
- 3 tablespoons of sea salt
- 1½ teaspoon of Shaoxing wine
- 3 tablespoons light soy sauce
- White sugar
- ½ teaspoon of sesame oil
- 24 fresh wonton wrappers

Directions

1. Dry-roast the Sichuan pepper with 3 teaspoons of sea salt in a heavy.
2. Once popping, remove, let cool.

3. Then, grind to a powder in a pestle and mortar.

4. Place chili flakes in a heatproof bowl.

5. Heat olive oil in a small heavy-based frying pan until it shimmering, pour the oil over the chili to release the flavor.

6. Stir, then let stand, uncovered, for 30 minutes.

7. Sieve the oil over a bowl, then, mix with remaining dressing ingredients.

8. Place the prawn meat, spring onion, ginger, and the remaining ingredients except for wonton, in a bowl.

9. Place in the refrigerator for 30 minutes covered.

10. Place a rounded teaspoon of prawn filling in the center of a wrapper.

11. Dip your finger in some water and moisten the bottom edge of the wrapper, then fold it in half.

12. Hold the wonton lengthways with the folded edge down.

13. Fold in half lengthways, then lightly moisten one corner of the folded edge.

14. Bring the two ends together with a twisting action, and seal.

15. Bring a large pan of water to the boil.

16. Then, drop the wontons, in batches, into the water, let cook for 2 minutes.

17. Serve and enjoy with the dressing, and sprinkled with Sichuan seasoning, prepared at the beginning.

Prawn and crab wontons

Ingredients

- 200g of white crabmeat
- 30 wonton wrappers
- 1 fresh red chili
- 2 tablespoons of oyster sauce
- 200g of peeled raw tiger prawns
- Groundnut oil
- Sweet chili sauce
- ½ tablespoon of sesame oil
- Corn flour
- 1 ginger
- 1 clove of garlic
- ½ bunch of chives

Directions

1. Combine ginger together with the garlic, chili, sliced chives, crabmeat, oyster sauce, sesame oil, and the prawn in a bowl. Mix to combine.
2. Lay the wonton wrappers on a clean work surface, cover with a damp.
3. Lightly dust a tray with corn flour.

4. Spoon 1 teaspoon of the filling onto the middle of a wrapper.
5. Brush the edges with a little water, then bring up over the filling, seal.
6. Place on the flour-dusted tray, then repeat with the remaining ingredients.
7. Pour boiling water into a saucepan over a medium-high heat.
8. Bring to the boil.
9. Cut out a circle of greaseproof paper so it fits snugly into a bamboo steamer, grease one side with oil, then place oil-side up into the steamer.
10. Add the wontons in a single layer, then place the basket on top of the pan, steam for 8 minutes covered.
11. Serve and enjoy with chili sauce.

Langoustines with lemon and pepper butter

Ingredients

- 100g of butter
- 1kg of fresh langoustines
- 2 teaspoons of coarse black pepper
- Olive oil
- 400 ml white wine
- 50g of fresh breadcrumbs
- 1 lemon
- 2 lemons

Directions

1. Combine the lemon zest, butter, black pepper, and a pinch of salt, keep for later.
2. Heat a grill to high.
3. Combine the langoustines and wine in a pan.
4. Bring to the boil, then lower the heat, let simmer for 5 minutes covered.
5. Place your langoustines, belly-side down, on a chopping board, cut in half lengthways, discarding the black vein in the tail.

6. Place, flesh-side up, on a baking tray, topping with the lemon butter, sprinkle over the breadcrumbs and drizzle with oil.
7. Grate the zest from 1 lemon into a bowl.
8. Place the lemon halves on the tray.
9. Let grill for 10 minutes.
10. Serve and enjoy sprinkled with zest and grilled lemon.

Szechuan sweet and sour prawns

Ingredients

- 150ml of unsweetened pineapple juice
- 300g of pineapple
- 1 tablespoon of low-salt soy sauce
- 1 red pepper
- 1 yellow pepper
- ½ bunch of fresh coriander
- 3 tablespoons of rice vinegar
- 2 cloves of garlic
- 2 fresh red chilies
- Sea salt
- 1 ginger
- ½ tablespoon of corn flour
- 24 peeled raw king prawns
- Groundnut oil

Directions

1. Preheat a large griddle pan over a high heat.
2. Add the pineapple for 4 minutes, turning occasionally.
3. Remove, let cool on a board.
4. Add sliced peppers to the griddle for about 3 minutes, turning halfway.

5. Bash the garlic together with the chilies, and a pinch of salt to a rough paste, in a pestle and mortar.
6. Add the ginger, then bash until broken down, combined.
7. Place the chili paste into a large bowl with the prawns and a splash of oil, mix.
8. Heat a lug of oil in a large non-stick frying pan over a medium-high heat.
9. Add the prawn mixture, let fry for 4 minutes.
10. Then, chop the cooled pineapple into bite-sized chunks.
11. In a bowl, combine the pineapple juice together with the vinegar, soy, corn flour, and a splash of water, add to the pan along with the chargrilled pineapple and peppers.
12. Bring to the boil, then, simmer over a low heat for about 2 minutes
13. Serve and enjoy with steamed rice.

Cooked oyster with burnt butter

Ingredients

- ½ of a lemon
- 800g of rock salt
- 40g of unsalted butter
- 8 rock oysters
- Tabasco sauce

Directions

1. Preheat the oven to the maximum heat.
2. Place the rock salt into an ovenproof frying pan.
3. Place the rock salt in the oven to preheat for around 20 minutes.
4. Then, place in the oysters on top, return the pan to the oven for 10 minutes.
5. Melt the butter in a frying pan over a medium heat, then cook for 3 minutes, or until the oyster turns to deep golden.
6. Add a few drops of Tabasco to taste.
7. Remove from heat, add a squeeze of lemon juice, swirling the pan until combined.
8. Put the pan to one side.

9. Insert an oyster knife in, then carefully lever it open.
10. Discard the oyster tops, then place the bottom shells with the oyster on a platter.
11. Serve and enjoy with a drizzle over the burnt butter.

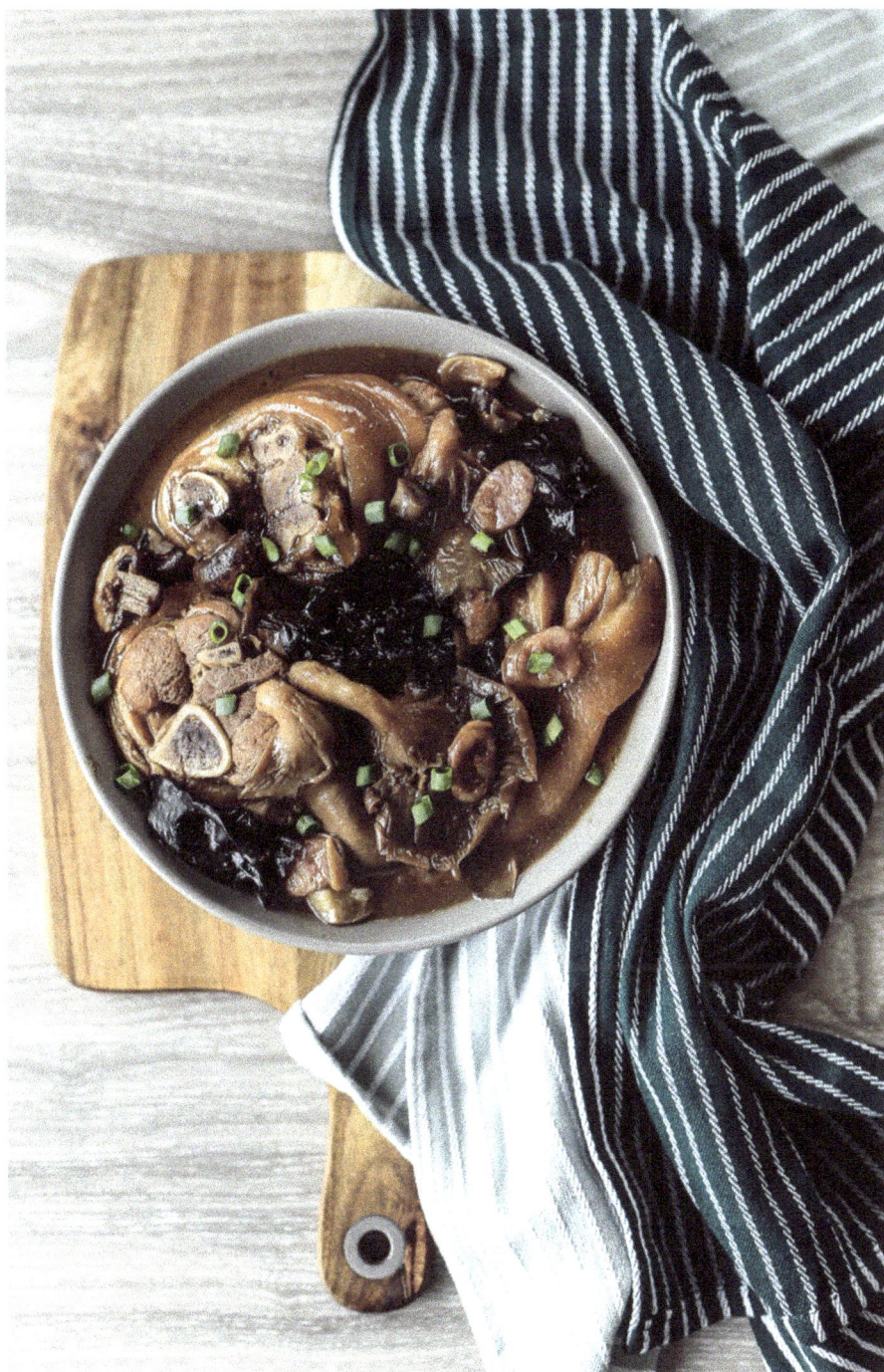

Cajun blackened fish steaks

Ingredients

- 2 level teaspoons of smoked paprika
- 4 x 200g of white fish fillets
- 1 teaspoon of cayenne pepper
- Lemon
- 10 sprigs of fresh thyme
- 2 tablespoons of olive oil
- 4 sprigs of fresh oregano
- 2 cloves of garlic

Directions

1. Bash the fresh herbs together with the garlic in a pestle and mortar until coarse paste forms.
2. Then, mix in the spices with bit of sea salt, black pepper, olive oil, and a squeeze of the juice of half the lemon, stir well.
3. Lightly score the skin of your fish in lines about 2cm apart.
4. Smear the rub all over both sides of the fish.
5. Place a pan over a medium-high heat.
6. Place the fish in the pan, skin side down, let cook for 4 minutes.

7. It will get quite smoky, so you might want to open a window.
8. Lower the heat, then, flip your fish over, and continue to cook for 4 minutes on the other side.
9. Cut the remaining lemon half and the second lemon into wedges.
10. Serve and enjoy the fish with salad and boiled potatoes dressed in good olive oil.

Barbecued langoustines with aioli

Ingredients

- 12 langoustines
- ½ clove garlic
- 1 teaspoon of sea salt
- Lemon juice
- 1 large egg yolk
- Sprigs fennel tops
- 1 teaspoon of Dijon mustard
- 300ml of extra virgin olive oil
- Freshly ground black pepper

Directions

1. To make the aioli, smash the garlic together with salt in a pestle and mortar.
2. Whisk the egg yolk with the mustard in a bowl, then adding olive oils to it bit by bit, the rest.
3. Add the smashed garlic with lemon juice, salt and pepper.
4. Lay the langoustines flat on a chopping board, with a sharp knife, saw through their shells lengthways.

5. Open them out in a butterfly style and flatten them down gently.
6. Season, then cook, cut-side down, across the bars on a hot Barbie for 2 minutes, then briefly on the other side.
7. Sprinkle with torn fennel tops.
8. Serve and enjoy with lemony aioli.

Creamy Cornish mussels

Ingredients

- 250ml of Cornish cider
- 600g of mussels
- 1 bunch of fresh chives
- 4 cloves of garlic
- 50g of clotted cream

Directions

1. Discard open mussels.
2. Place a large deep pan on a high heat.
3. Then, pour in 1 tablespoon of olive oil, add garlic with chives, and cider.
4. Bring to a fast boil, add the mussels with the clotted cream, cover and leave for 4 minutes, shaking occasionally.
5. When all the mussels have opened, they are done. Discard any closed ones.
6. Taste the sauce, and adjust the seasoning with sea salt and black pepper.
7. Sprinkle over the remaining chives.
8. Serve and enjoy.

Pesto mussels and toast

Ingredients

- 50ml of white wine
- 70g of pesto
- 160g of fresh or frozen peas
- 2 thick slices of whole meal bread
- 500g of mussels
- 200g of baby courgettes
- 200g of ripe mixed-color cherry tomatoes
- 2 sprigs of fresh basil

Directions

1. Put a large pan on a medium-high heat.
2. Toast the bread as the pan heats up, turn when golden.
3. Remove the toast, spread one quarter of the pesto on each slice.
4. Turn on the heat under the pan to full heat.
5. Place in the mussels.
6. Stir in the remaining pesto, together with the courgettes, tomatoes, and peas.
7. Add the wine let cover and steam for 4 minutes, shaking the pan occasionally.

8. When all the mussels have opened and are soft, they are done.

9. Divide the mussels, vegetables, and juices between 2 large bowls.

10. Pick over the basil leaves and serve with the pesto toasts on the side.

11. Enjoy.

Mussels with Guinness

Ingredients

- 1 fresh bay leaf
- ½ a bunch of fresh thyme
- 1 shallot
- 250ml of Guinness
- 2 cloves of garlic
- 2 rashers of smoked bacon
- 1kg of mussels
- 50ml of double cream
- ½ a bunch of fresh flat-leaf parsley
- 1 knob of unsalted butter

Directions

1. In a pan, melt the butter and sweat the shallot with the garlic and bacon for 5 minutes.
2. Add half of the herbs, together with the bay and a pinch of sea salt and black pepper.
3. Then, add the mussels, then the Guinness.
4. Let boil, then lower the heat, let steam for 5 minutes covered.
5. Stir in the cream and remaining herbs.
6. Taste, and adjust the seasoning.

7. Serve and enjoy with bread.

Shellfish and cider stew

Ingredients

- 1 tablespoon of unsalted butter
- 4 ripe plum tomatoes
- 3 leeks
- 600g of clams
- 600g of mussels
- 3 shallots
- 6 razor clams
- ½ a bunch of fresh flat-leaf parsley
- 500ml of organic fish stock
- 750ml of cider
- 1 teaspoon of tomato purée
- 6 langoustines
- 3 tablespoons of double cream

Directions

1. Start by melting the butter in a large pan over a low heat.
2. Gently fry the leeks together with the shallots, tomatoes, and parsley until soft.
3. Season, then add the stock with cider.

4. Raise the heat, let the liquid boil for 10 minutes, until reduces slightly.

5. Warm a large serving bowl.

6. Add the langoustines, cover for 3 minutes.

7. Then add the razor clams. Cook for a further 2 minutes while covered.

8. Add the mussels together with the clams.

9. Stir gently, then, add another splash of cider, cover, let cook for a further 5 minutes, or until the mussels and clams have opened.

10. Transfer the shellfish to the warmed serving bowl and put the sauce back on the heat.

11. Add the cream together with the tomato purée, stir well to combine.

12. Pour the sauce over the shellfish in the bowl.

13. Serve and enjoy with crusty bread.

Simple baked cod with tomatoes

Simple baked cod is flavorful due to the garlic, lemon, and herbs used typically basil.

It is a perfect Mediterranean Sea diet for dinner or lunch.

Ingredients

- salt, pepper and chili flakes to taste
- 3 tablespoons of olive oil
- ¼ cup of basil leaves torn
- 2 cups of cherry
- 3 garlic cloves rough chopped
- 2 lb. of cod fillets
- 1 lemon – zest and slices

Directions

1. Begin by preheating your oven ready to 400°F.
2. Pour the olive oil in a baking dish .
3. Scatter the garlic cloves.
4. Add the tomatoes with lemon slices, toss and pus to one side.

5. Pat dry the fish, place in the baking dish , turn to coat each side with oil.

6. Spread out the tomato garlic mixture and nestle in the fish.

7. Make sure tomatoes on the sides, lemons underneath.

8. Season all with salt , pepper and chili flakes.

9. Let bake for 10 minutes, scatter with lemon zest.

10. Continue to bake for 5 more minutes.

11. Add the torn basil leaves, tossing with the warm tomatoes.

12. Garnish every piece of fish with a wilted basil leaf.

13. Serve and enjoy immediately.

Roasted salmon with braised lentils

Ingredients

- 7 garlic cloves, finely minced
- 1 tablespoon of fresh thyme
- 2 teaspoons of whole-grain mustard
- 2 cups of French Green Lentils
- Fresh thyme sprigs for garnish
- 2 teaspoons of lemon zest
- 2 bay leaves
- 5 sprigs of fresh thyme
- ¼ cup of sherry wine
- 3 teaspoon of salt
- pepper to taste
- 2 lbs. of salmon
- 1 onion, diced
- 1 cup of diced celery
- 5 tablespoon of olive oil
- 1 cup of diced carrot
- 4 cups of veggie

Directions

1. Preheat heat oven to 325F.
2. Pat dry the salmon.
3. Combine garlic with thyme, whole grain, lemon zest, olive oil, salt and pepper in a small bowl.
4. Brush a little marinade on the bottom sides of salmon.
5. Then, place on parchment -lined sheet pan .
6. Spoon the remaining over top, to form a thin layer. Set aside.
7. Bake salmon in the preheated oven for 15 minutes or so.
8. Heat oil in a large sauté pan over medium heat.
9. Add onion together with the celery and carrots.
10. Stir for 5 minutes, lower the heat, continue to cook for more 5 more minutes.
11. Add the garlic and lentils.
12. Cook for 2 minutes while stirring.
13. Add the wine. Let this cook-off, about 2 minutes.
14. Pour in the stock, salt , and mustard, and stir until combined, let simmer.
15. Add the bay leaves and thyme sprigs, cover and gently simmer on low heat for 30 minutes.
16. Taste and adjust accordingly.
17. Serve and enjoy.

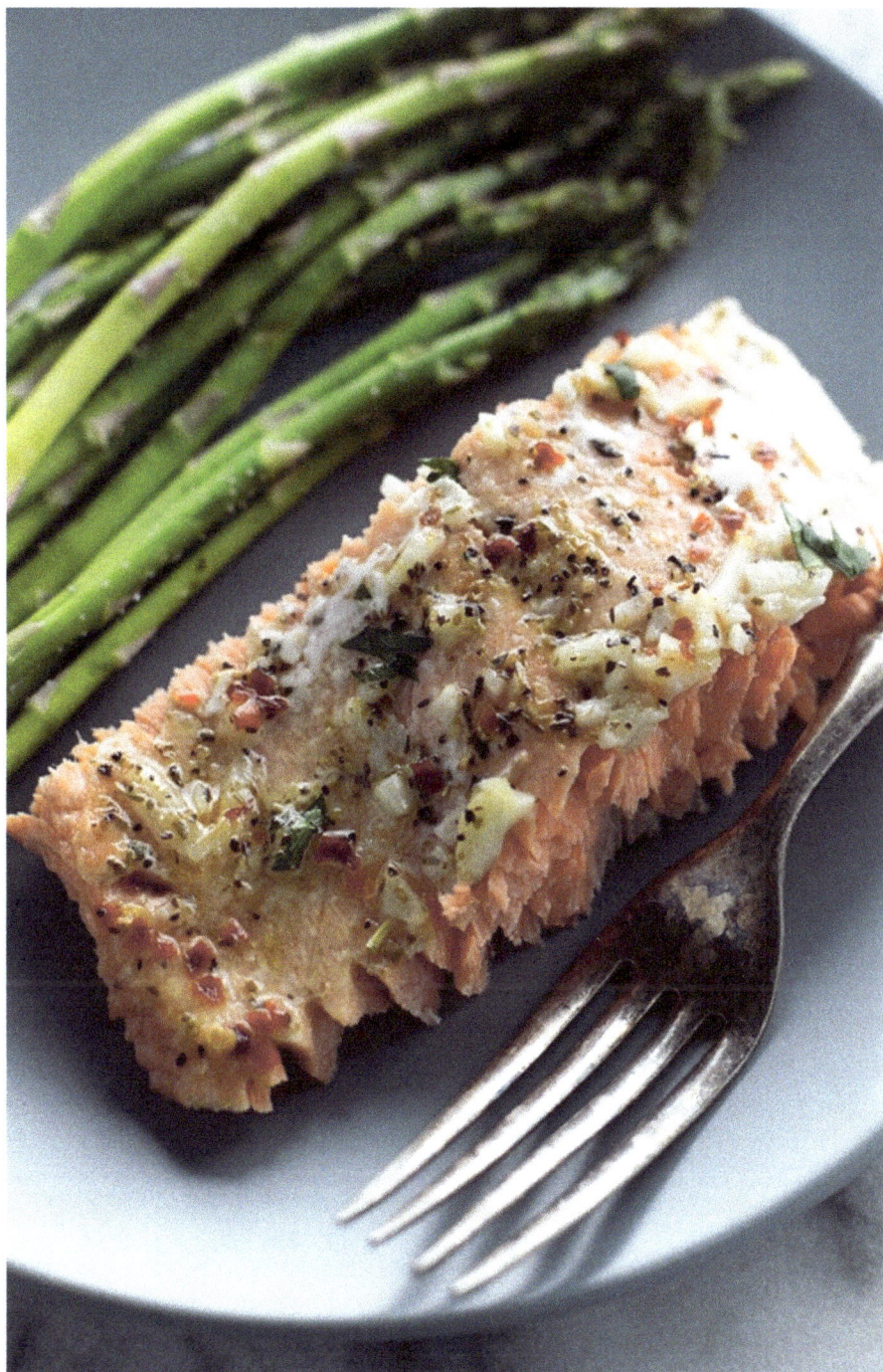

www.ingramcontent.com/pod-product-compliance
Lightning Source LLC
Chambersburg PA
CBHW050755030426
42336CB00012B/1828